Praise for 5:2 DIET FOR V⅃

*"Here is all the information you need
to lose those extra pounds."*

"Excellent book for vegetarian 5:2 dieters."

*"This little book has simple soups,
easy salads and light meals
that are just a little bit different."*

"Useful little book."

*"Tasty recipes which make it easy to stick to
the restricted calorie allowance."*

*"Fasting day meals are a great idea.
With herby scrambled egg on toast
coming in at a mere 150 calories,
it all felt very doable."*

*"Broccoli and orange soup, aubergine chilli
and shakshouka are some of the unusual dishes
I can't wait to try."*

Joy Bounds is a writer and lives in Suffolk. Her interests, which are reflected in her writing, are history and the issues which affect women.

This is Joy's first cookery book. She has been a vegetarian for over forty years, and loves to try new dishes. She has travelled widely, and likes to introduce foods and flavors from other countries into her recipes. She also loves a challenge, and in this book she has taken many well-known and well-loved dishes, and recreated them to fit into the low calorie-count required by the 5:2 diet.

You can find out more about her at www.joybounds.co.uk or on Facebook at Joy Bounds, Suffolk Writer.

Joy Bounds

5:2 DIET

for

VEGETARIANS

4 weeks of calorie-counted meals & recipes
for fast days

Luscious Books

Published by Luscious Books Ltd 2016
Morwellham, Down Park Drive, Tavistock, PL19 9AH, Great Britain

ISBN 978-1-910929-04-9

Copyright © Joy Bounds 2016
Cover image © Vesna Cvorovic | 123rf.com

This book was originally published as a Kindle ebook
by Luscious Books Ltd 2014

A CIP catalogue record for this book is available from the British Library.

www.lusciousbooks.co.uk

Contents

∿ Meal plans & recipes ∿

Disclaimer

The information provided in this book is not a substitute for professional medical care, advice or guidance from a doctor or other suitably qualified healthcare professional. It cannot be warranted that any information included in this book will meet your particular health or medical requirements.

It is very important that you seek medical advice from a doctor or other suitably qualified healthcare professional if you have any concerns or questions about your health and diet.

The author of this book is not a medical doctor. This book merely contains information and recipes that she has found useful in managing her own diet.

The 5:2 diet is generally suitable for people in good general health. You should not follow the diet if

* you have type 1 diabetes
* you are pregnant, trying to get pregnant or are breastfeeding
* you have or have had an eating disorder
* you are already very thin/underweight
* you are a child or a teenager
* you are a frail elderly person

If your doctor or other suitably qualified healthcare professional thinks that you should not fast, please follow his/her advice. The aim of this diet is to improve wellbeing, not to make it worse.

Introduction

There's an ideal state, perhaps, in which we're so in tune with our world that we eat just what our body needs to keep healthy. However, most of us are not in that state. We use food for comfort, to compensate us for tough experiences, for reward. Many of us are too easily tempted by foods that we know are not particularly good for us, or we eat much more than we actually need.

Over the years lots of people have come up with different kinds of diets and eating plans to help us control our weight and feel better. Perhaps you have tried some of them. What makes the 5:2 diet different is that it doesn't require as much self-discipline as many other diets. You only watch your food intake two days a week, and the other five days you can eat normally.

I started the 5:2 diet a couple of years ago and at that time there weren't that many suitable vegetarian recipes available. I started to develop my own recipes and discovered — quite unexpectedly — that following a new eating plan renewed my interest in all my cookbooks. I also became fascinated by the challenge of getting every last benefit out of my meagre calorie allowance on the fasting days.

This book contains my fasting day meal ideas and recipes for vegetarians and anyone interested in vegetarian dishes. I hope that this recipe book will give you a start on some new, healthy, low-calorie dishes that will inspire you to carry on with the 5:2 diet long after the initial four weeks are up!

The 5:2 diet

The 5:2 diet, as we know it today, was introduced by Dr Michael Mosley in a TV documentary *Horizon: Eat, Fast, Live Longer* in August 2012. It's based on a range of scientific experiments into the health benefits of intermittent fasting. (If you're interested in finding out more about these studies, have a look at Michael Mosley and Mimi Spencer's book *The Fast Diet* and Brad Pilon's website, www.bradpilon.com.)

Following the 5:2 diet means fasting on two non-consecutive days a week and eating sensibly on the other five. It's up to you to decide which days you want to fast.

Fasting days don't equate to complete abstinence from food: women are allowed to eat 500 kcal a day and men 600 kcal. It doesn't matter where the calories come from as long as the limit is not exceeded. As calories add up very quickly, one way to maximize the amount of food you can eat is to have drinks that contain no or virtually no calories, such as water, herbal and fruit teas, black tea or black coffee.

Although the diet is considered only to be taking place during the two fasting days a week, in some ways the success of the eating plan as a weight-losing tool also depends on what we do on the five normal days. Normal eating days are meant to be normal — as long as 'normal' doesn't mean lots of pies, pastries, chocolate and cakes! If you want to lose weight, try eating healthily during the non-fasting days too. Two fasting days and five days of sensible eating will usually result in weight loss of about a pound a week.

How to use this book

Starting any new programme of eating can be confusing, and I hope that this book will help to avoid that.

This book gives you a 4-week eating plan and recipes for fasting days. It's designed to make the 5:2 diet easy to follow:

* There are separate meal plans to suit both men and women.
* The calories have been counted so you don't have to.
* All the meals are easy to prepare.
* Most of the meals will keep in a fridge for a few days or will freeze well, so you can prepare some meals in advance if you want to.
* There is a wide range of vegetable and salad dishes to choose from so you won't get bored.

When Dr Mosley introduced his version of the 5:2 diet, he recommended eating breakfast in the morning, and dinner as late in the day as possible. Although a long 'fasting window' is supposed to have enhanced health benefits, many people find it difficult to eat only two meals a day.

This book gives you an alternative: divide your daily calorie intake into three, or even four, by having three meals or three meals and a snack. Although this means that some of the health benefits of not eating for several hours may be lost, it's still an effective way of implementing the 5:2 diet. In fact, following normal mealtime routines can make it easier to stick to the diet in the long run — and that is ultimately the main goal.

In my meal plan, I have listed 'breakfast', 'light meal' and 'main meal' options as well as some additional snacks. You can eat the meals in whichever order you like during your fasting day. It's best not to swap the recipes between different days, though, as your overall calorie intake may exceed the daily allowance.

For each fasting day, I have included a small amount of milk. You can use it with your tea or coffee. If you don't use milk in your tea or coffee, drink it as it is or add it to your cereal or even a soup.

I hope you find this book useful in reaching your weight loss goals and in feeling better in yourself.

Useful tips

Most people are able to incorporate the low-calorie days into their week without feeling anything but a few hunger pangs — after all, we can't cut our daily calorie intake by 75% without feeling hungry. However, most people are surprised by how insignificant these hunger pangs become after the first few days. One amazing thing is that if you are hungry at 7pm, it isn't going to get worse and worse all night long. After a short while, it will simply disappear, may recur briefly a few hours later, only to go again.

Diversion is a good tool for managing hunger pangs. Take your attention away from your stomach, for example by absorbing yourself in an activity you like, and you will find that the fasting day goes quickly. The knowledge that the following day you can eat normally again can also help.

Fasting days may also feel strange because the portion sizes that we are allowed to eat are often smaller than what we're used to. You can fool your brain a little by using smaller plates and bowls: this will make you think that you're having a plateful or a bowlful of food, even if your portions are not as large.

When you're eating, slow down and take your time to savor the flavors of your meal. Often we eat in a hurry and without really tasting our food, and subsequently, end up eating more than we really need. Now is a good time to learn to listen to your body.

Some people have reported having a slight headache when starting fasting. This can often be avoided by drinking more water than usual. Until the body gets used to the change in eating habits, it might be wise to avoid hard physical work on the first few low-calorie days. Generally speaking, however, many people feel that their concentration and general energy levels become enhanced as a result of intermittent fasting.

When you start fasting, monitor yourself carefully, and consult your doctor or other suitably qualified healthcare professional if you feel any adverse effects.

About measurements

I have used metric units (grams and millilitres), imperial measures (ounces and fluid ounces) and US cups throughout this book.

Be aware that mixing the different measuring units in one recipe may lead to an unsuccessful result, so decide which system you want to use and stick to that. If possible, however, I would recommend using metric measures as they are more precise than imperial units or cups.

It's important to have good measuring tools, such as digital scales and measuring cups. It's best to use teaspoons and tablespoons that are specifically meant for cooking and baking purposes as the spoons used in everyday life tend to be smaller. The accurate volume of a teaspoon is 5 ml and a tablespoon is 15 ml. Also, always use level measures.

About calorie counting

Calorie counting is perhaps not quite as exact a scientific process as we like to think. Most calorie-counting books or computer programs will give similar values for basic foodstuffs (for example, a bag of flour), but as soon as the product is used for something more complex (for example, a loaf of bread), then variations begin to show.

Because of this, there may be a variation of a few calories either way in each meal plan. This isn't something to worry about, but when you go shopping, it's best to choose the lowest-calorie products available.

About ingredients and kitchen equipment

Basic kitchen equipment is all you need to make the recipes in this book. It's useful, however, to have solid and/or non-stick saucepans so that food can be cooked in as little oil as possible.

As there are so many calories in fat and oil, it has been used sparingly. Ideally, only use a couple of spurts of oil spray/cooking spray per dish. If you don't have it, a little pastry or basting brush will help to coat the pan with a minimum amount of oil.

Many of the recipes use herbs and/or spices. A range of these is necessary to get maximum flavor from the dishes, so make sure that your store cupboard has a good supply. Fresh herbs can enhance a simple dish greatly, but if it's not possible to have many of these, parsley and basil are good to have fresh, since these do not dry well. Otherwise, dried herbs are perfectly good.

Throughout the book, I have used 'vegetable stock', without being specific. Normally, I would prefer to use home-made stock, but as this is almost impossible to calorie-count, a vegetable stock cube/ bouillon cube is the best option. Compare a few different brands in the supermarket and buy the one with the least calories.

MEAL PLANS
&
RECIPES

WEEK 1 — DAY 1 MEAL PLAN

Women (495 kcal)

Breakfast (p. 21)
Fruit with yogurt and honey — women's portion (115 kcal)

Light Meal (p. 22)
Broccoli and orange soup (150 kcal)

Main Meal (p. 24)
Leek omelette — women's portion (175 kcal)

Additionally
100 ml (3 ½ fl oz) scant ½ cup skimmed milk/skim milk (35 kcal)
2 dried apricots (20 kcal)

Men (595 kcal)

Breakfast (p. 21)
Fruit with yogurt and honey — men's portion (135 kcal)

Light Meal (p. 22)
Broccoli and orange soup (150 kcal)

Main Meal (p. 24)
Leek omelette — men's portion (245 kcal)

Additionally
100 ml (3 ½ fl oz) scant ½ cup skimmed milk/skim milk (35 kcal)
3 dried apricots (30 kcal)

WEEK 1 — DAY 1 RECIPES

Fruit with yogurt and honey

Women (115 kcal)

30 g (1 oz) ¼ cup raspberries

30 g (1 oz) ¼ cup blueberries

4 grapes

4 tbsp fat-free natural yogurt

2 tsp honey

Men (135 kcal)

30 g (1 oz) ¼ cup raspberries

30 g (1 oz) ¼ cup blueberries

4 grapes

6 tbsp fat-free natural yogurt

2 tsp honey

1. Cut the grapes in half.

2. Mix the grapes, raspberries and blueberries in a breakfast bowl.

3. Spoon the yogurt on top.

4 Drizzle the honey over the yogurt and fruit.

Broccoli and orange soup

Broccoli and orange is an unusual combination, but a delicious one. The orange adds lightness and a distinctive flavor to the dish.

3 portions (1 portion 150 kcal)

1 small (100 g/3 ½ oz) onion

1 tbsp vegetable oil

350 g (12 oz) 2 cups broccoli florets

2 tbsp plain wholemeal flour/whole wheat flour

600 ml (25 fl oz) 2 ½ cups vegetable stock (use stock/bouillon cubes or buy ready-made stock)

1 orange

salt and black pepper to taste

1. Peel and chop the onion.

2. If you haven't bought broccoli florets in a bag, but a whole broccoli, prepare it now: cut out the tough central stalk and cut the rest of the broccoli into small florets. You can also use the smaller stalks if you like.

3. Measure the vegetable stock and put it into a jug. If you're using stock/bouillon cubes, mix them into hot water.

4. Thinly peel the orange. Discard half of the peelings and cut the rest into small pieces. Then squeeze the juice of the orange into a cup.

5. In a saucepan, heat the oil, add the onion and cook it on a low heat until it becomes translucent. Stir every now and then.

6. When the onion is cooked, sprinkle the flour into the saucepan and cook the mixture for 1 minute, stirring constantly.

7. Pour the stock slowly into the saucepan, stirring all the time. Raise the heat under the pan and stir until the soup comes to the boil and thickens a little.

8. Add the broccoli and the orange peelings into the pan. Cover the pan with a lid and cook for about 20 minutes, until the broccoli florets are tender. Season with salt and pepper.

9. Take the saucepan off the heat. Remove a few broccoli florets and put them aside.

10. Pour the soup into a blender or blend it with a hand blender until it becomes smooth.

11. Return the soup to the pan, add the broccoli florets and mix in the juice of the orange.

12. Reheat the soup until it comes to the boil. Taste and add more seasoning if need be.

13. Divide the soup into 3 portions and put one portion into a bowl. You can keep the rest of the soup in a fridge for a few days or freeze it for another fasting day.

Leek omelette

Women (175 kcal)	**Men (245 kcal)**
100 g (3 ½ oz) 1 cup leeks	*100 g (3 ½ oz) 1 cup leeks*
25 g (1 oz) 2 tbsp frozen sweet corn	*25 g (1 oz) 2 tbsp frozen sweet corn*
¾ tbsp light/medium fat cream cheese	*¾ tbsp light/medium fat cream cheese*
10 g (scant ½ oz) 2 tsp blue cheese	*10 g (scant ½ oz) 2 tsp blue cheese*
½ tsp dried thyme or ½ tbsp fresh thyme	*½ tsp dried thyme or ½ tbsp fresh thyme*
salt and black pepper to taste	*salt and black pepper to taste*
1 medium egg	*2 medium eggs*
1 tbsp cold water	*1 tbsp cold water*
3 sprays oil spray/cooking spray	*3 sprays oil spray/cooking spray*

1. Cut the leeks into the small slices.

2. Steam the leeks: you can do this by placing them in a steaming basket over boiling water for about 10 minutes, or by placing them in a non-metallic bowl with a small amount of boiling water and microwaving them for 4-5 minutes.

3. In the middle of the cooking period, stir in the frozen sweet corn and continue to cook.

4. Drain the vegetables and cool for a few minutes. Then put them into a mixing bowl.

5. Add the cream cheese, blue cheese, thyme and some salt and pepper into the bowl and mix.

6. Break the egg(s) into a separate mixing bowl and add the water. Lightly beat the mixture together until fully combined.

7. Heat a small frying pan and coat it with some oil spray/cooking spray. When the pan is moderately hot, pour in the egg(s) and swirl about to create an even layer.

8. Continue cooking the egg(s). When the mixture has almost set, spread the vegetables and cheese on top. Turn down the heat and leave the omelette to cook for a couple of minutes until the topping is heated through.

9. Fold over the omelette and place on a plate to serve.

Variation

Instead of leek, you can make this omelette with 50 g (2 oz) scant ½ cup of fresh asparagus.

WEEK 1 — DAY 2 MEAL PLAN

Women (500 kcal)

Breakfast (p. 29)
Herby scrambled egg on toast — women's portion (150 kcal)

Light meal (p. 30)
Colorful salad (125 kcal)

Main meal (p. 32)
Chilli (190 kcal)

Additionally
50 ml (2 fl oz) scant ¼ cup skimmed milk/skim milk (18 kcal)
4 medium (65 g/2 oz) strawberries (17 kcal)

Men (600 kcal)

Breakfast (p. 29)
Herby scrambled egg on toast — men's portion (225 kcal)

Light meal (p. 30)
Colorful salad (125 kcal)

Main meal (p. 32)
Chilli (190 kcal)

Additionally
50 ml (2 fl oz) scant ¼ cup skimmed milk/skim milk (18 kcal)
4 medium (65 g/2 oz) strawberries (17 kcal)
A tangerine (25 kcal)

WEEK 1 — DAY 2 RECIPES

Herby scrambled egg on toast

Women (150 kcal)	Men (225 kcal)
1 medium egg	1 medium egg
1 tbsp water	1 tbsp water
salt and black pepper to taste	salt and black pepper to taste
1 tbsp fresh herbs of your choice or 1 tsp dried mixed herbs	1 tbsp fresh herbs of your choice or 1 tsp dried mixed herbs
2 sprays oil spray/cooking spray	2 sprays oil spray/cooking spray
1 small slice (30 g/1 oz) wholemeal bread/whole wheat bread	2 small slices (60 g/2 oz) wholemeal bread/whole wheat bread
scrape low-fat vegetable oil spread	scrape low-fat vegetable oil spread

1. Put the egg and water into a small mixing bowl and gently beat together. Mix in the salt, pepper and herbs.

2. Put a couple of sprays of oil spray/cooking spray into a small non-stick saucepan. Pour the egg mixture in and heat gently. Stir frequently to prevent sticking. When the scrambled egg is ready, take it off the heat.

3. Toast the bread. Scrape as little low-fat spread on top as possible.

4. Pile the scrambled egg onto the toast and serve.

Colorful salad

This is a delicious, fresh-tasting salad, with crunchy pine nuts for texture.

1 portion (125 kcal)

50 g (2 oz) generous ¼ cup cucumber

50 g (2 oz) generous ¼ cup courgette/zucchini

50 g (2 oz) generous ¼ cup melon of your choice

1 spring onion/scallion

1 tbsp lemon juice

½ tsp olive oil

salt and black pepper to taste

2 small tomatoes

4 radishes

A handful of fresh basil leaves or ½ tsp dried mixed herbs

2 tbsp pine nuts

1. Thinly slice the cucumber and courgette/zucchini (about a coin's thickness) and cut the slices into quarters. Place the pieces in a mixing bowl.

2. Peel and deseed the melon. Slice it into similar sized pieces as the cucumber. Add the melon pieces into the bowl.

3. Finely chop the spring onion/scallion. Add it together with the lemon juice and oil into the mixing bowl and toss everything together. Season to taste.

4. Cut the tomatoes into slices and radishes into as thin slices as you can.

5. Put these slices onto a shallow dish and sprinkle with fresh basil leaves or dried mixed herbs.

6. Spoon the contents of the mixing bowl on top of the tomatoes and radishes.

7. Heat a saucepan over a medium heat. Add the pine nuts and lightly brown them. Shake them occasionally. (There's no need to use any oil for this.)

8. Sprinkle the pine nuts on top of the salad and serve.

Chilli

This is a classic dish with many variations. It's traditionally made with kidney beans, but I prefer the lighter cannellini or haricot/ navy beans.

Although it's a simple dish, it's not a quick one to make as the flavors need time to develop. Therefore, it's best to leave it to simmer for as long as possible.

2 portions (1 portion 190 kcal)

½ medium (100 g/3 ½ oz) aubergine/eggplant

1 small (100 g/3 ½ oz) onion

1 clove garlic

50 g (2 oz) ½ cup celery

75 g (2 ½ oz) scant ½ cup red pepper/bell pepper

good pinch dried red chillies or 1 green chilli

½ tbsp olive oil

1 tsp cumin

pinch smoked paprika

200 g (7 oz) scant 1 cup chopped tomatoes from a tin/can

1 tbsp tomato purée/paste

115 g (4 oz) ½ cup cannellini, haricot/navy or kidney beans from a tin/can (drained weight)

200ml (7 fl oz) scant 1 cup vegetable stock (use stock/bouillon cubes or buy ready-made stock)

salt and black pepper to taste

+ 1 tbsp fat-free natural yogurt per portion

1. Start by cooking the aubergine/eggplant. You can do this either in a microwave or by steaming it. If you prefer to use the microwave, prick the skin of the aubergine/eggplant a few times with a sharp knife and microwave on high for 1 minute. If you'd like to steam your aubergine, place it in a steaming basket on top of a pan of boiling water for 15 minutes. When you have cooked the aubergine/eggplant, it should be a little bit soft but not mushy. Allow it to cool.

2. Peel and chop the onion. Finely chop the celery and garlic.

3. Remove the pith and seeds from the red pepper/bell pepper and chop it into pieces. If you are using a fresh green chilli instead of dried chillies, remove the pith and seeds from that as well and chop it finely.

4. Measure the vegetable stock and put it into a jug. If you're using a stock/bouillon cube, mix it into hot water. Set the jug aside for the time being.

5. Heat the oil in a large saucepan. Add the onions and celery and cook on a low heat without browning for 10 minutes. Stir every now and then.

6. Add the red pepper/bell pepper, stir and leave to cook for further 5 minutes. Mix occasionally.

7. Stir in the garlic, chilli, cumin and smoked paprika. Cook for 2 minutes.

8. Cut the aubergine/eggplant into 1 cm (½ inch) cubes and add to the pan with the tomatoes, stock and tomato purée/paste. Season and simmer gently for 20 minutes until the vegetables are cooked.

9. Drain the beans and add them into the saucepan. Simmer the chilli on a very low heat for about 1 hour without a lid, until it

When you're eating, slow down and take your time to savor the flavors of your meal.

Now is a good time to learn to listen to your body.

has a rich, thick consistency. If it becomes a little dry, stir in a few tablespoonfuls of boiling water. Check the seasoning and add more salt and pepper as required.

10. Divide the chilli into 2 portions. Put 1 portion into a bowl and top with 1 tablespoon of yogurt.

You can keep the remaining portion in the fridge for a couple of days or you can freeze it and eat it on another fasting day.

WEEK 2 — DAY 1 MEAL PLAN

Women (500 kcal)

Breakfast (p. 39)
Boiled egg with bread (145 kcal)

Light meal (p. 40)
Mushroom and chestnut soup (145 kcal)

Main meal (p. 42)
Green and red warm salad (170 kcal)

Additionally
50 ml (2 fl oz) scant ¼ cup skimmed milk/skim milk (18 kcal)
1 cracker with a scrape of of yeast extract (for example, Marmite or Vegemite) (22 kcal)

Men (599 kcal)

Breakfast (p. 39)
Boiled egg with bread (145 kcal)

Light meal (p. 40)
Mushroom and chestnut soup (145 kcal)

Main meal (p. 42)
Green and red warm salad (170 kcal)

Additionally
100 ml (3 ½ fl oz) scant ½ cup skimmed milk/skim milk (35 kcal)
2 crackers with a scrape of yeast extract (for example, Marmite or Vegemite) (44 kcal)
A small apple (60 kcal)

WEEK 2 — DAY 1
RECIPES

Boiled egg with bread

1 portion (145 kcal)

1 medium egg

1 small slice (30 g/1 oz) wholemeal bread/whole wheat bread

scrape low-fat vegetable oil spread

1. Place the egg in a saucepan and cover it with cold water. Bring the water to the boil and boil the egg for 3 minutes if you like a soft-boiled egg or for 5 minutes if you prefer a hard-boiled one.

2. If you like, toast the bread. Lightly spread the slice of bread with the low-fat spread and cut it into four pieces.

3. Take the egg out of the pan and put it into an egg-cup, cracking the shell lightly to stop it cooking further. Serve it with the bread slices.

Mushroom and chestnut soup

2 portions (1 portion 145 kcal)

15 g (½ oz) ⅓ cup dried porcini mushrooms

500 ml (18 fl oz) 2 cups light vegetable stock (use stock/bouillon cubes or buy ready-made stock)

1 clove garlic

60 g (2 oz) ⅔ cup fresh mushrooms

100 g (3 ½ oz) generous ¾ cup vacuum-packed chestnuts

1 tsp oil

1 tbsp fresh thyme or 1 tsp dried thyme

2 tbsp fresh parsley

salt and black pepper to taste

+ 1 tbsp fat-free yogurt per portion

1. Measure the vegetable stock, put it into a small saucepan and heat it. Please note: in this recipe it's better to make the stock weaker than you would normally as rehydrating the mushrooms will strengthen the stock.

2. Take the saucepan off the heat. Rehydrate the porcini mushrooms in the hot stock for 10-15 minutes (according to your packet's instructions).

3. Meanwhile, finely chop the garlic, fresh mushrooms and chestnuts.

4. Heat the oil gently in another (larger) saucepan and fry the garlic, thyme and parsley for 2-3 minutes. Stir constantly and be careful not to burn the garlic.

5. Add the fresh mushrooms. Continue cooking, stirring occasionally, for 5 minutes.

6. Chop the rehydrated porcini mushrooms. Add them as well as the stock into the pan. Bring the liquid to the boil and simmer for 5 minutes.

7. Add the chestnuts and continue to simmer for another 10 minutes. Season to taste.

8. Take the saucepan off the heat and take out a few slices of mushrooms.

9. Pour the soup into a blender or blend it with a hand blender until it becomes smooth.

10. Pour the soup back into the saucepan and mix in the mushrooms you took out earlier.

11. Divide the soup into 2 portions and put 1 portion into a bowl. Let it cool slightly, then stir in 1 tablespoon of yogurt and serve. You can keep the remaining portion in the fridge for a few days.

Green and red warm salad

This deceptively simple dish is made quite special by the roast tomato sauce. It is best served warm, or at room temperature, rather than hot.

2 portions (1 portion 170 kcal)

1 medium (150 g/5 ½ oz) red pepper/bell pepper

3 medium (260 g/9 oz) tomatoes

2 cloves garlic

½ tsp dried mixed herbs

1 tsp oil

200 g (7 oz) 2 generous cups green beans/string beans (fresh or frozen)

1-2 tsp balsamic vinegar

salt and black pepper to taste

20 g (¾ oz) 2 tbsp light feta cheese

1 tbsp fresh basil or parsley

Croutons

1 small slice (30 g/1 oz) white bread

½ tbsp vegetable oil

1. Pre-heat the oven to 200C/400F/Gas Mark 6.

2. Remove the pith and seeds from the red pepper/bell pepper and halve them.

3. Cut each tomato horizontally into two halves.

4. Take a roasting dish and place the pepper halves in it facing down.

5. Put in the roasting dish the tomato halves facing up. Coat the tomatoes with the oil and dried mixed herbs. Tuck in the garlic cloves in between them (there's no need to peel them at this stage).

6. Put the roasting dish in the oven and bake for 20-25 minutes, until the pepper skins are beginning to blacken.

7. While the vegetables are roasting, cut the green beans/string beans into 5 cm (2 inch) pieces and the feta cheese into small cubes. Set them aside.

8. Next prepare the croutons: cut the bread into small cubes and put them into an oven-proof dish. Add the oil and toss them so they become evenly coated.

9. When the roasted vegetables are ready, take them out of the oven and set aside to cool.

10. Turn the oven down to 150C/300F/Gas Mark 2.

11. Put the red pepper/bell pepper halves into a plastic food bag (this will help the skins to come off easily later).

12. Once the oven temperature is lower, place the croutons in the oven and bake for 7-8 minutes. Take them out of the oven, turn them over with a spoon or spatula and return them to the oven for another 7-8 minutes.

13. While the croutons are baking, boil the green beans/string beans in water (salted to taste) for 5-10 minutes, until they are tender.

Many people feel that

their **concentration** and

energy levels become

enhanced

as a result of intermittent fasting.

14. While the beans are boiling, remove the skins from the red pepper/bell pepper halves and discard them. Cut the peppers into strips. Set aside.

15. Scoop the tomato pulp from their skins and put the pulp into a mixing bowl. Discard the skins.

16. Squeeze the garlic gloves from their skins. Discard the skins. Slice the garlic thinly and add to the tomato pulp.

17. Add the balsamic vinegar, salt and pepper. Stir vigorously or blend.

18. When the beans are cooked, take them off the heat and drain them.

19. When the croutons are ready, take them out of the oven.

20. Divide the dish into 2 portions: Place the beans on 2 serving plates. Scatter the strips of red pepper/bell pepper, the skins of the tomatoes and the cubed feta over the top.

21. Spoon over the tomato dressing and sprinkle with fresh basil or parsley. Serve 1 portion immediately with half of the croutons scattered on top, and save the other portion and eat it within a couple of days (keep it covered in the refrigerator, storing the croutons separately, and bring it up to room temperature before serving).

WEEK 2 — DAY 2
MEAL PLAN

Women (500 kcal)

Breakfast (p. 49)
Porridge with blueberries (140 kcal)

Light meal (p. 50)
Salad bowl (155 kcal)

Main meal (p. 52)
Ratatouille (150 kcal)

Additionally
50 ml (2 fl oz) scant ¼ cup skimmed milk/skim milk (18 kcal)
1 small tangerine (25 kcal)
50 g (2 oz) ⅓ cup melon (12 kcal)

Men (596 kcal)

Breakfast (p. 49)
Porridge with blueberries (140 kcal)

Light meal (p. 50)
Salad bowl (155 kcal)

Main meal (p. 52)
Ratatouille (150 kcal)

Additionally
75 ml (2 ¾ fl oz) ⅓ cup skimmed milk/skim milk (26 kcal)
1 banana (100 kcal)
1 tangerine (25 kcal)

WEEK 2 — DAY 2 RECIPES

Porridge with blueberries

1 portion (140 kcal)

30 g (1 oz) ⅓ cup porridge oats

250 ml (9 fl oz) 1 cup cold water

30 g (1 oz) ⅓ cup blueberries

1. Put the porridge oats and water into a saucepan and bring slowly to the boil. Simmer for 3-4 minutes until the oats are soft and they have absorbed the water. Stir from time to time.

2. Pour the porridge into a bowl and scatter the blueberries on top.

You can also make the porridge in a microwave:

1. Put the porridge oats and water into a microwaveable dish and microwave on full for about 2 minutes. The exact time depends on how powerful your microwave is. If it looks like the porridge is about to bubble over, take the porridge out of the microwave and give it a stir. Then continue. The porridge is ready when the oats are soft and they have absorbed the water.

2. Pour the porridge into a bowl and scatter the blueberries on top.

Salad bowl

This salad has a delicious combination of tastes and textures and it's also full of colour.

1 portion (155 kcal)

25 g (1 oz) ½ cup lettuce

50 g (2 oz) generous ¼ cup cucumber

4 cherry tomatoes

4 radishes

25 g (1 oz) ¼ cup mushroom

25 g (1 oz) ¼ cup carrot

25 g (1 oz) 2 tbsp green or red pepper/bell pepper

1 spring onion/scallion

1 tsp rice vinegar

fresh basil

salt and black pepper to taste

10 g (¼ oz) 1 tbsp light feta cheese

Croutons

½ medium slice (20 g/¾ oz) white bread

½ tsp vegetable oil

1. Start by making the croutons. Pre-heat the oven to 150C/300F/Gas Mark 2.

2. Cut the bread into small cubes and put it into an oven-proof dish. Add the oil and toss them so they become evenly coated.

3. Place the croutons in the oven and bake for 7-8 minutes. Take them out of the oven, turn them over with a spoon or spatula and return them to the oven for another 7-8 minutes.

4. While the croutons are baking, chop the lettuce, cut the cucumber into ½ cm (¼ inch) cubes, halve the tomatoes, finely slice the radishes and mushrooms, grate the carrot and finely chop the pepper and spring onion/scallion.

5. Put all the vegetables into a shallow serving bowl and mix them thoroughly.

6. Drizzle over the rice vinegar, fresh basil, salt and pepper. Toss everything together.

7. Cut the feta cheese into small cubes. Sprinkle it over the salad.

8. Arrange the croutons on top of the salad and serve.

Variation

If you don't have radishes, you can use 25 g (1 oz) ¼ cup finely chopped celery instead.

You can also use other fresh or dried herbs instead of basil.

Ratatouille

Ratatouille is a traditional vegetable dish from the Provence region of France. It benefits from simmering for a while, so try to leave time for the flavors to develop. The addition of pasta, while not normally seen within the traditional dish, goes well, and makes it more substantial.

2 portions (1 portion 150 kcal)

1 small (100 g/3 ½ oz) onion

½ medium (75 g/2 ½ oz) red pepper/bell pepper

1 clove garlic

½ medium (150 g/5 oz) aubergine/eggplant

1 medium (125 g/4 ½ oz) courgette/zucchini

½ tbsp olive oil

200 g (7 oz) 1 cup chopped tomatoes from a tin/can

up to 300 ml (18 fl oz) 1 ¼ cups vegetable stock (use stock/ bouillon cubes or buy ready-made stock)

2 tbsp mixed fresh herbs or 1 tsp dried mixed herbs

scant ¼ tsp smoked paprika

salt and black pepper to taste

½ tbsp tiny pasta shapes (for example, orzo or stellette)

10 g (¼ oz) 1 tbsp parmesan cheese

fresh parsley to garnish

1. Chop the onion. Remove the pith and seeds from the red pepper/bell pepper and cut it into pieces. Chop the garlic finely and the aubergine/eggplant into 1 cm (½ inch) cubes. Thinly slice the courgette/zucchini.

2. Heat the oil in a large saucepan and add the onion. Sweat it on a low heat, stirring every now and then, until it becomes translucent. This will take about 10 minutes.

3. Stir in the red pepper/bell pepper and garlic. Continue to sweat them for another 5 minutes, mixing them occasionally.

4. Stir in the aubergine/eggplant, put a lid on the pan and continue to sweat the vegetables for 5 more minutes.

5. Mix in the courgette/zucchini and cook with lid on for a further 5 minutes.

6. While the vegetables are gently simmering, measure the vegetable stock and put it into a jug. If you're using a stock/bouillon cube, mix it into hot water. Set the jug aside.

7. The vegetables should now be softening. Season with salt and pepper.

8. Stir in the tomatoes, stock, smoked paprika and mixed herbs and allow to simmer in the covered pan on a low heat for at least 20 minutes — up to 1 hour would be ideal.

9. Add the pasta shapes and cook gently for a further 15 minutes with no lid on the pan, stirring occasionally. If it looks like the ratatouille is getting dry, add more stock or a little water.

10. While the ratatouille is cooking, grate the parmesan cheese. Place 4 small piles of it on a baking tray. Grill/Broil these gently until they have melted and formed little crispy discs.

11. Divide the ratatouille as well as the parmesan discs into 2 portions. Put 1 portion into a bowl, top it with the parmesan discs and garnish with some parsley. You can freeze the remaining portion (excluding the parmesan discs) and eat it on another fasting day.

WEEK 3 — DAY 1 MEAL PLAN

Women (490 kcal)

Breakfast (p. 57)
Weetabix with fruit (110 kcal)

Light meal (p. 58)
Butternut squash soup (125 kcal)

Main meal (p. 60)
Shakshouka (185 kcal)

Additionally
100 ml (3 ½ fl oz) scant ½ cup skimmed milk/skim milk (35 kcal)
8 grapes (35 kcal)

Men (591 kcal)

Breakfast (p. 57)
Weetabix with fruit (110 kcal)

Light meal (p. 58)
Butternut squash soup (125 kcal)

Main meal (p. 60)
Shakshouka (185 kcal)

Additionally
100 ml (3 ½ fl oz) scant ½ cup skimmed milk/skim milk (35 kcal)
9 grapes (40 kcal)
2 crackers with 10 g (¼ oz) 2 tbsp blue cheese (74 kcal)
2 dried apricots (22 kcal)

WEEK 3 — DAY 1 RECIPES

Weetabix with fruit

1 portion (110 kcal)

1 Weetabix

50 ml (2 fl oz) scant ¼ cup skimmed milk/skim milk

50 g (2 oz) ⅓ cup melon

50 g (2 oz) generous ½ cup frozen or fresh raspberries

1. Put the Weetabix into a bowl.

2. Peel and chop the melon. Scatter them and the raspberries over the Weetabix.

3. Add milk and serve.

Butternut squash soup

3 portions (1 portion 125 kcal)

½ medium (300 g/10 oz) butternut squash

2 tsp vegetable oil

1 clove garlic

1 small (100 g/3 ½ oz) onion

1 tbsp fresh thyme leaves or 1 tsp dried thyme

good pinch chilli powder

60 g (2 oz) ⅓ cup carrot

1 small (100 g/3 ½ oz) potato

600 ml (20 fl oz) 2 ¼ cups vegetable stock (use stock/bouillon cubes or buy ready-made stock)

salt and black pepper to taste

fresh parsley

+ 1 tbsp fat-free yogurt per portion

1. Peel and deseed the butternut squash. Cut it into 2 cm (1 inch) chunks.

2. Chop the onion and garlic. Slice the carrot. Peel and cut the potato into small pieces.

3. Put the oil into a saucepan and heat it on a low heat. Add the onions and cook gently for 5 minutes.

4. Add the thyme, chilli powder, garlic, carrot slices, potato pieces and butternut squash chunks. Stir thoroughly. Cover the pan with a lid and cook the vegetables for 5 minutes.

5. Measure the vegetable stock and put it into a jug. If you're using a stock/bouillon cube, mix it into hot water.

6. Add the stock into the pan, bring to the boil and simmer with the lid on for about 20 minutes until the vegetables are soft.

7. Take the pan off the heat and purée the soup in a blender or with the help of a hand blender.

8. Taste and season with salt and pepper as needed.

9. If the soup doesn't feel hot enough, put it back into the saucepan and reheat.

10. Divide the soup into 3 portions and serve one portion in a bowl with 1 tablespoon of yogurt and a sprinkle of parsley. You can freeze the remaining portions.

Shakshouka

This dish has many versions in different countries, but the essential ingredients are red peppers/bell peppers and eggs. In this version, Middle-Eastern style, the combination of herbs and spices gives it a great flavor.

1 portion (185 kcal)

35 g (1 ¼ oz) ¼ cup onion

125 g (4 ½ oz) ⅔ cup red or orange peppers/bell peppers

125 g (4 ½ oz) ¾ cups tomatoes

scant ¼ tsp cumin seeds

1 tsp olive oil

1 tsp tomato purée/paste

1 tbsp hot water

1 tsp sugar (preferably brown)

1 bay leaf

1 tbsp mixed fresh coriander/cilantro, parsley and thyme or 1 tsp mixed dried herbs

pinch cayenne pepper

scant ¼ tsp allspice

salt and black pepper to taste

1 medium egg

1. Chop the onion. Remove the pith and seeds from the pepper/bell pepper and cut it into strips. Chop the tomatoes.

2. Dry-fry the cumin seeds by placing them in a small frying pan and heating them on a medium heat for about 2 minutes, until they release their scent. Stir them occasionally.

3. Add the oil and the chopped onion into the pan, and fry on a low heat for about 5 minutes, stirring every now and then to prevent sticking.

4. Add the peppers into the pan and cook on a medium heat for about 10 minutes, until softened. Stir frequently.

5. Mix the tomato purée/paste with 1 tablespoon of hot water.

6. Add the sugar, bay leaf, herbs, cayenne pepper, allspice, tomatoes and tomato purée/paste into the pan, and season with salt and pepper.

7. Reduce the heat and let the mixture simmer with the lid on the pan for about 10 minutes. Stir occasionally. Add a little boiling water if necessary to create a thick sauce-like consistency. Remove the bay leaf, and check seasoning.

8. Create a 'well' in the mixture, and break the egg into it.

9. Cover the pan and leave it for 7-10 minutes on a low heat until the egg is set. Try to resist the temptation to keep lifting the lid as the egg will not cook if the steam is lost!

10. Spoon the egg and the vegetable mixture carefully onto a plate. Sprinkle with parsley and a grind of black pepper and serve.

WEEK 3 — DAY 2 MEAL PLAN

Women (495 kcal)

Breakfast (p. 65)
Melba toast with cream cheese and fruit (152 kcal)

Light meal (p. 66)
Tomato, cucumber and mozzarella salad (160 kcal)

Main meal (p. 68)
Polenta with mushroom ragout — women's portion (150 kcal)

Additionally
50 ml (2 fl oz) scant ¼ cup skimmed milk/skim milk (18 kcal)
1 plum (15 kcal)

Men (597 kcal)

Breakfast (p. 65)
Melba toast with cream cheese and fruit (152 kcal)

Light meal (p. 66)
Tomato, cucumber and mozzarella salad (160 kcal)

Main meal (p. 68)
Polenta with mushroom ragout — men's portion (182 kcal)

Additionally
50 ml (2 fl oz) scant ¼ cup skimmed milk/skim milk (18 kcal)
1 cracker with yeast extract (for example, Marmite or Vegemite)
(25 kcal)
1 small apple (60 kcal)

WEEK 3 — DAY 2 RECIPES

Melba toast with cream cheese and fruit

1 portion (152 kcal)

4 small (15 g/½ oz) melba toasts

1 tbsp medium fat cream cheese

1 small banana

50 g (2 oz) ¼ cup strawberries

1. Slice the banana thinly and put it into a mixing bowl.

2. Mix in the cream cheese.

3. Spread the mixture evenly over the melba toasts.

4. Cut the strawberries into quarters and place on top of the melba toasts.

Tomato, cucumber and mozzarella salad

A simple set of ingredients are made special by marinating the mozzarella, and adding a couple of strong flavors to the salad. Dried tomatoes in oil are high in calories, so use the dried ones that need rehydrating.

This salad is served with a cracker. It doesn't matter what kind of cracker you have as long as it's 20-25 kcal.

1 portion (160 kcal)

2 halves (10 g/¼ oz) sun-dried tomatoes (the dry variety, not in oil)

1 tsp vegetable oil

1 tsp balsamic vinegar

1 small clove garlic

salt and black pepper to taste

30 g (1 oz) 1 ½ tbsp low-fat mozzarella cheese

10 medium (100 g/3 ½ oz) cherry tomatoes

50 g (2 oz) ⅓ cup cucumber

1 tbsp fresh basil or parsley (or 1 tsp dried mixed herbs)

1 cracker to serve

1. Rehydrate the sun-dried tomatoes according to the packet instructions.

2. Peel and crush the garlic.

3. Put it into a mixing bowl with the oil, vinegar, salt and pepper.

4. Cut the mozzarella into small pieces and put it into the bowl. Mix thoroughly with the other ingredients and leave to marinade for about 10 minutes.

5. While the mozzarella is marinating, cut the cherry tomatoes into quarters and the cucumber into batons.

6. Put the tomatoes and cucumber onto a plate and sprinkle with fresh basil or parsley.

7. Drain the rehydrated tomatoes, cut them into small pieces and sprinkle them over the tomatoes and cucumber.

8. Spoon the mozzarella onto the salad and pour over the remaining marinade.

9. Serve with the cracker.

Variation

Instead of sun-dried tomatoes, use 3 finely sliced spring onions/scallions or 3 olives in brine.

Polenta with mushroom ragout

Polenta/cornmeal is a staple of North Italy. In this recipe the porcini mushrooms add depth of flavor, but if none are available, use a few more fresh mushrooms and some well-flavored stock.

Women (150 kcal)	Men (182 kcal)
10 g (scant ½ oz) scant ¼ cup dried porcini mushrooms	*10 g (scant ½ oz) scant ¼ cup dried porcini mushrooms*
40 g (1 ½ oz) ¼ cup polenta/ cornmeal	*40 g (1 ½ oz) ¼ cup polenta/ cornmeal*
10 g (¼ oz) ¾ tbsp grated parmesan cheese	*20 g (¾ oz) 1 ½ tbsp grated parmesan cheese*
salt and black pepper to taste	*salt and black pepper to taste*
very small (50 g/2 oz) onion (or shallot)	*very small (50 g/2 oz) onion (or shallot)*
1 clove garlic	*1 clove garlic*
150 g (5 ½ oz) 1 ½ cups fresh mushrooms (white or chestnut or a mixture)	*150 g (5 ½ oz) 1 ½ cups fresh mushrooms (white or chestnut or a mixture)*
½ tsp + ¼ tsp oil	*½ tsp + ¼ tsp oil*
½ tbsp fresh thyme or ½ tsp dried thyme	*½ tbsp fresh thyme or ½ tsp dried thyme*
3 sprays oil spray/cooking spray	*3 sprays oil spray/cooking spray*
fresh parsley to serve	*fresh parsley to serve*

1. Rehydrate the porcini mushrooms according to the instructions on the packet.

2. Cook the polenta/cornmeal according to packet instructions.

Remove it from the heat. Beat into the mixture the parmesan cheese, and season with salt and pepper.

3. Lay out the polenta/cornmeal on a plate or wooden board to create a rectangle about 1 cm (¼ inch) thick. Leave it to cool.

4. Finely slice the onion. Peel and crush the garlic. Slice the fresh mushrooms.

5. Heat ½ teaspoon of oil in a pan and gently cook the onion for about 10 minutes, adding the garlic for the final minute.

6. Add the fresh mushrooms, and leave to cook gently for about 10 minutes, stirring occasionally to ensure they release their juices.

7. Drain the rehydrated porcini mushrooms, retaining the stock. Cut the mushrooms into small pieces and add them into the pan.

8. Also add the thyme, and season the mushroom mixture with salt and pepper.

9. Sieve the retained mushroom stock to remove any grit, and add 75 ml (3 fl oz) ⅓ cup of that into the pan.

10. Stir everything together, and leave to simmer without a lid for 10 minutes, allowing the stock to boil down a little. Add more salt and pepper if desired.

11. Using a pastry brush, paint the polenta/cornmeal with ¼ teaspoon of oil, and cut it roughly into 4 triangles or slices.

12. Spray a frying pan with oil spray/cooking spray and fry the polenta /cornmeal gently on both sides until just coloured.

13. Put the polenta /cornmeal on a plate and top with the ragout.

14. Sprinkle with parsley and serve.

WEEK 4 — DAY 1 MEAL PLAN

Women (500 kcal)

Breakfast (p. 73)
Muesli with apple — women's portion (135 kcal)

Light meal (p. 74)
Green soup (115 kcal)

Main meal (p. 76)
Roasted cauliflower with tahini sauce (185 kcal)

Additionally
100 ml (3 ½ fl oz) scant ½ cup skimmed milk/skim milk (35 kcal)
6 cherries (30 kcal)

Men (600 kcal)

Breakfast (p. 73)
Muesli with apple — men's portion (205 kcal)

Light meal (p. 74)
Green soup (115 kcal)

Main meal (p. 76)
Roasted cauliflower with tahini sauce (185 kcal)

Additionally
100 ml (3 ½ fl oz) scant ½ cup skimmed milk/skim milk (35 kcal)
7 cherries (35 kcal)
100 g (3 ½ oz) ¾ cup melon of your choice (25 kcal)

WEEK 4 — DAY 1 RECIPES

Muesli with apple

Women (135 kcal)

20 g (¾ oz) 2 tbsp muesli

1 small (100 g/3 ½ oz) apple

50 ml (1 ¾ fl oz) scant ¼ cup skimmed milk/skim milk

Men (205 kcal)

40 g (1 ½ oz) 4 tbsp muesli

1 small (100 g/3 ½ oz) apple

50 ml (1 ¾ fl oz) scant ¼ cup skimmed milk/skim milk

1. Pour the muesli into a bowl.

2. Finely chop or grate the apple and add with the blueberries to the muesli.

3. Add milk and serve.

Green soup

This is a marvellously healthy, bright green soup which is easy to prepare.

3 portions (1 portion 115 kcal)

1 medium (100 g/3 ½ oz) onion

2 sticks (100 g/3 ½ oz) celery

120 g (4 ½ oz) ¾ cup courgette/zucchini

½ large (140 g/5 oz) potato

½ tbsp vegetable oil

600 ml (18 fl oz) 2 cups vegetable stock (use stock/bouillon cubes or buy ready-made stock)

100 g (3 ½ oz) ⅔ cup peas (fresh and shelled, or frozen)

handful fresh basil and/or parsley (or 1 tsp dried herbs)

salt and black pepper to taste

100 g (3 ½ oz) 2 cups fresh or scant ½ cup frozen spinach

1. Chop the onion and celery into small pieces. Cut the courgette/zucchini and the potato into 1 cm (½ inch) cubes.

2. Heat the oil in a saucepan. Add the onion and celery and cook on a low heat for about 5 minutes, stirring every now and then.

3. Add the courgette/zucchini, stir and continue to cook for another 5 minutes. Mix occasionally.

4. Measure the vegetable stock and put it into a jug. If you're using a stock/bouillon cube, mix it into hot water.

5. Add the potato cubes and the stock into the saucepan, bring the liquid to the boil, cover the saucepan with a lid and let the soup simmer on a low heat for 10 minutes.

6. Stir in the peas and bring the soup back to a simmer.

7. Add half of the fresh basil/parsley and season with salt and pepper.

8. Add the spinach and stir thoroughly to mix it in. Keep the soup simmering.

9. Remove the saucepan off the heat. Take a small ladleful of the soup and put it into a bowl and set it aside. Purée the rest of the soup in a blender or with the help of a hand blender.

10. Pour the soup back into the saucepan, including the ladleful that wasn't puréed. Add the rest of the basil/parsley. Reheat the soup.

11. Check the seasoning and add more salt and pepper if need be. Divide the soup into 3 portions. Serve 1 portion immediately. Keep the rest of the portions in the fridge for a few days or freeze them.

Roasted cauliflower with tahini sauce

This is a Lebanese-style dish. Roasting gives cauliflower an interesting, nutty flavor, and the unusual sauce makes for a satisfying, tasty meal, completed by a little side salad.

1 portion (185 kcal)

200 g (7 oz) ½ cup cauliflower

1 tsp olive or sunflower oil

juice of 1 lemon

salt and black pepper to taste

1 clove garlic

2 tsp fresh parsley or coriander/cilantro

2 ½ tsp light tahini paste

1-2 tsp water

1 medium (100 g/3 ½ oz) tomato

few chives (or basil leaves) or ½ tsp mixed herbs

salt and black pepper

1. Pre-heat the oven to 200C/400F/Gas mark 6.

2. Cut the cauliflower into bite-sized florets and wash them. Don't dry them afterwards as it's better to leave them a little wet when they go in the oven. Place the florets on a baking tray/pan.

3. Cut the lemon into halves. Put one half aside and drizzle the juice of the other half as well as the oil over the cauliflower. Season with salt and pepper, and toss everything together.

4. Roast the cauliflower florets in the oven for 15 minutes. Take them out of the oven, turn them over with a spoon or spatula and return them to the oven for another 10-15 minutes, until they are cooked and slightly browned. If they look a little dry, add a sprinkle of water and a couple of sprays of oil spray/cooking spray. The cauliflower should still have a bite to it after it's been roasted, and a few charred edges will add to the flavor. When the cauliflower is ready, take it out of the oven and let it rest in the baking tray/pan.

5. Crush the garlic clove and chop the fresh herbs.

6. Take the lemon half that you had put aside earlier and squeeze its juice into a cup.

7. Take a small mixing bowl and mix the tahini, half of the lemon juice (leave the rest in the cup) and the crushed garlic in it. Add the chopped herbs.

8. Add 1-2 teaspoons of water into the mixture to make it into a smooth, thick but still pourable paste.

9. Chop the tomato into small chunks, and place it in a small mixing bowl.

10. Snip the chives into tiny pieces (or chop the basil leaves) and mix them in with the chopped tomato.

11. Mix the remaining lemon juice into the tomato and herb mixture. Season to taste.

12. To serve, put the cauliflower onto a plate and spoon over the sauce. Serve the tomato salad on the side.

WEEK 4 — DAY 2 MEAL PLAN

Women (500 kcal)

Breakfast (p. 81)
Toast and marmalade (135 kcal)

Light meal (p. 82)
Crackers, raw vegetables and dip — women's portion (145 kcal)

Main meal (p. 84)
Aubergine/eggplant with tofu and noodles — women's portion (165 kcal)

Additionally
100 ml (3 ½ fl oz) scant ½ cup skimmed milk/skim milk (35 kcal)
5 medium (75 g/2 ½ oz) strawberries (20 kcal)

Men (595 kcal)

Breakfast (p. 81)
Toast and marmalade (135 kcal)

Light meal (p. 82)
Crackers, raw vegetables and dip — men's portion (170 kcal)

Main meal (p. 84)
Aubergine/eggplant with tofu and noodles — men's portion (235 kcal)

Additionally
100 ml (3 ½ fl oz) scant ½ cup skimmed milk/skim milk (35 kcal)
5 medium (75 g/2 ½ oz) strawberries (20 kcal)

WEEK 4 — DAY 2 RECIPES

Toast and marmalade

1 portion (135 kcal)

1 small slice (35 g/1 ¼ oz) wholemeal bread/whole wheat bread

1 tsp low-fat vegetable oil spread

1 tsp marmalade

1. Toast the bread.

2. Lightly spread it with the low-fat spread.

3. Spread marmalade on top and serve.

Crackers, raw vegetables and dip

This is an easy light meal for a lunchbox, or a day when there's not much time to cook. There are many crackers on the market, but choose ones which have 20-25 kcal in each.

Women (145 kcal)	Men (170 kcal)
2 crackers	3 crackers
10 g (¼ oz) 2 tbsp blue cheese	10 g (¼ oz) 2 tbsp blue cheese
15 g (½ oz) 2 inch piece carrot	15 g (½ oz) 2 inch piece carrot
3 cherry tomatoes	3 cherry tomatoes
3 radishes	3 radishes
30 g (1 oz) scant ¼ cup green pepper/bell pepper	30 g (1 oz) scant ¼ cup green pepper/bell pepper
1 medium stick (50 g/2 oz) celery	1 medium stick (50 g/2 oz) celery
2 tbsp thick fat-free yogurt	2 tbsp thick fat-free yogurt
1 tsp light mayonnaise	1 tsp light mayonnaise
1 tbsp fresh herbs (for example, chives, parsley and/or thyme) or ½ tsp dried mixed herbs	1 tbsp fresh herbs (for example, chives, parsley and/or thyme) or ½ tsp dried mixed herbs

1. Spread the crackers with the blue cheese.

2. Peel the carrot and cut it into small batons.

3. Halve the cherry tomatoes.

4. Quarter the radishes.

5. Cut the pepper into slices.

6. Cut the celery into small batons or chunks.

7. Make the dip by mixing the yogurt, mayonnaise and herbs together in a small a ramekin or cup.

8. Place the crackers and vegetables on a plate and serve with the dip.

Variation

Instead of using the listed salad ingredients — that is, carrot, cherry tomatoes, radishes, green pepper/bell pepper or celery — you can replace any one of them with 30 g (1 oz) ⅓ cup mushrooms or 40 g (1 ½ oz) ¼ cup cucumber.

Aubergine/eggplant with tofu and noodles

This Japanese-style meal packs quite a tasty punch given the small number of calories, the acidic marinade contrasting with the other soothing ingredients.

Women (165 kcal)	Men (235 kcal)
1 small (125 g/4 ½ oz) aubergine/eggplant	1 small (125 g/4 ½ oz) aubergine/eggplant
1 small clove garlic	1 small clove garlic
1 tsp ginger	1 tsp ginger
1 spring onion/scallion	1 spring onion/scallion
¼ tsp oil	¼ tsp oil
1 tsp mirin	1 tsp mirin
1 tsp rice vinegar	1 tsp rice vinegar
1 tsp soy sauce (preferably light)	1 tsp soy sauce (preferably light)
25 g (1 oz) ⅓ cup dried noodles	45 g (1 ¾ oz) scant ⅔ cup dried noodles
50 g (2 oz) ½ cup tofu	50 g (2 oz) ½ cup tofu
1 tsp miso paste	1 tsp miso paste
50 ml (2 fl oz) ¼ cup boiling water	50 ml (2 fl oz) ¼ cup boiling water

1. Cut the aubergine/eggplant in half and peel it. You can either cook it in a microwave or steam it. If you steam it, place it in a steaming basket on top of a pan of boiling water for 15 minutes. To microwave it, cook it on high power for 2 minutes, and then

leave to stand for a further 2 minutes. The aubergine/eggplant should be soft and cooked through.

2. Leave the aubergine/eggplant to cool for a few minutes, then cut or tear it with your fingers into short strips.

3. Peel and crush the garlic clove. Peel the ginger and chop it finely. Chop the spring onion/scallion into small pieces.

4. Make the marinade: place the oil, mirin, rice vinegar, soy sauce, garlic and ginger into a shallow mixing bowl and stir well to combine.

5. Add the aubergine/eggplant strips into the marinade. Keep on turning them every now and again while you continue to prepare the rest of the meal.

6. Cook the noodles according to the packet instructions, then drain them.

7. While the noodles are cooking, drain the tofu and cut into ½ cm (¼ inch) cubes.

8. Dissolve the miso paste in 50 ml (2 fl oz) ¼ cup of boiling water to make a broth.

9. Place the tofu, noodles, miso broth and spring onion/scallion in a saucepan or small wok and heat through.

10. Keeping the aubergine/eggplant aside, add any remaining marinade into the saucepan and mix.

11. Serve the contents of the saucepan in a shallow bowl, and place the aubergine/eggplant strips on top.

Recipe index

Luscious Books is an
independent publishing house
specialising in wellbeing titles.

Find more cookbooks for special diets at

www.lusciousbooks.co.uk

15673356R00055

Printed in Poland
by Amazon Fulfillment
Poland Sp. z o.o., Wrocław